A SIMPLIFIED DIET COOKBOOK FOR ULCER

The Ultimate Ulcer-Friendly Recipes to Manage Symptoms

TABLE OF CONTENT

CHAPTER ONE

ULCER TYPES

Ulcers are open sores that can occur on internal and external parts of the body. They can be mild or serious. There are seven common types of ulcers: peptic, esophageal, arterial, diabetic foot, venous, genital, and mouth. Depending on the location of the ulcer, symptoms can include pain, nausea, heartburn, or itching. Treatment can include antibiotics, acid reducers, antiviral drugs, surgery, or lifestyle changes.

Peptic ulcers

There are two main types of peptic ulcers.

- Gastric ulcers develop in the stomach.

- Duodenal ulcers develop in the upper part of the small intestine, which is called the duodenum.

Causes

There are two main causes of peptic ulcers.

- Bacterial infection: Infection with the bacterium Helicobacter pylori (H. pylori) can cause inflammation and damage to your stomach and duodenum linings, resulting in ulcers.

- Nonsteroidal anti-inflammatory drugs (NSAIDs): NSAIDs, including aspirin and ibuprofen, are typically used to treat pain. Frequent use of NSAIDs can cause ulcers because these drugs make your stomach and duodenum more vulnerable to stomach acid.

Contrary to popular belief, stress and spicy foods do not cause ulcers. However, certain foods may worsen an ulcer that is already present.

Symptoms

Some common symptoms of peptic ulcers include:

- stomach pain, usually in the upper abdomen

- fullness or bloating

- heartburn

- nausea

- vomiting

Esophageal ulcers

Esophageal ulcers form in the esophagus, which is the tube that connects your throat to your stomach. When the inner lining of the esophagus is damaged, an ulcer forms.

Causes

The most common cause of esophageal ulcers is gastroesophageal reflux disease (GERD), or acid reflux. This condition occurs when stomach acid backs up into the esophagus. Stomach acid wears away the lining of the esophagus, causing ulcers.

Other causes of esophageal ulcers include:

- frequent vomiting

- the use of medications that irritate the esophagus

- infections

- the consumption of liquids rich in acid, such as caffeinated drinks and alcohol

- smoking

Symptoms

The symptoms of esophageal ulcers include heartburn, difficulty swallowing, chest pain, a sensation of food not going down right or getting stuck in your throat, nausea, vomiting or excessive saliva

Diagnosis

As with peptic ulcers, your doctor may perform an EGD to diagnose esophageal ulcers. They may also perform a barium-contrast esophagram. During this procedure, you will swallow a liquid containing barium sulfate. This liquid will coat the esophagus so that the lining is clearly visible on an X-ray.

Treatment

Treatment for esophageal ulcers mainly focuses on treating the underlying cause. If you have an ulcer caused by GERD, your doctor will likely prescribe PPIs or H_2 blockers. H_2 blockers are medications that reduce the amount of acid produced by the stomach, providing temporary relief. If an infection caused your ulcer, a doctor could prescribe antibiotics or antiviral medications. If a medication irritates your esophagus, you may need to stop taking it.

Making lifestyle changes, such as quitting smoking and drinking fewer acid-rich liquids, may be beneficial in healing and preventing esophageal ulcers. It is also helpful to maintain an appropriate diet.

Arterial ulcers

Arterial ulcers, also called ischemic ulcers, occur when there is an insufficient blood supply to the lower extremities. They frequently occur on the feet and lower legs. An open wound forms when your skin and tissue do not receive adequate blood supply.

Causes

The causes of arterial ulcers include:

- atherosclerosis, which is a condition wherein your arteries narrow because of plaque accumulation

- high blood pressure

- minor injuries that heal slowly

- diabetes

- kidney failure

- vasculitis, which causes your blood vessels to become inflamed

Symptoms

Arterial ulcers typically appear as symmetrical open wounds on your lower legs or feet. They can be brown, black, yellow, or gray. These ulcers typically do not bleed, but they are extremely painful.

Other symptoms of arterial ulcers include increased pain at night, cool, shiny skin surrounding the wound, leg hair loss or faint pulse in the extremity

Diagnosis

To diagnose an arterial ulcer, a doctor will examine your medical history and symptoms. They may also perform certain tests, including:

- Buerger test: This test involves analyzing how well blood flows to your extremities. You will lie flat on a bed, raise your leg to a 45-degree angle for 1 minute, and then lower it below the bed. The color of your foot in these positions can indicate insufficient blood flow.

- Transcutaneous oximetry: This measures the oxygen content of the skin around the wound. If the test shows low oxygen content, it can indicate arterial insufficiency.

- Ankle-brachial pressure index (ABPI): This is a measurement of the blood pressure in your arm and your ankle.

- Capillary refill time: This measures how long it takes for the blood vessels in your skin surface to fill with blood after they are pressed.

Treatment

Treatment for arterial ulcers involves addressing the underlying cause. For example, if high blood pressure caused an arterial ulcer, you may need to make some lifestyle and diet changes. If the wound shows signs of an infection, such as swelling or discharge, your doctor may prescribe oral antibiotics.

In some cases, doctors may use skin grafting to cover the wound. The affected extremity may also need surgical revascularization, which involves either bypassing narrowed vessels or reopening them. This procedure will promote healing by restoring blood flow to the area.

Diabetic foot ulcers

Diabetic foot ulcers are common among people with uncontrolled diabetes. Researchers estimate that 15–25% of people with diabetes will develop a diabetic foot ulcer. These ulcers typically develop on the bottom of the foot.

Causes

The main causes of diabetic foot ulcers include:

- inadequate foot care

- peripheral vascular disease, which is a condition wherein the blood vessels in the lower extremities become narrowed and restrict blood flow

- neuropathy, which is a condition wherein nerve damage causes pain, weakness, or numbness

- atypical blood sugar levels

Symptoms

A diabetic foot ulcer will appear as an open wound, commonly on the bottom of your foot. The wound may have the following characteristics; drainage, potentially with an odor, tissue discoloration, commonly black or brown, calluses, swelling, blisters or pain

Diagnosis

To diagnose a diabetic foot ulcer, your doctor may perform tests such as:

- swabbing the wound or taking a deep tissue sample to look for signs of infection

- blood tests to check certain substance levels, including blood sugar levels

- scans and probes to check for bone involvement

Treatment

To treat diabetic foot ulcers, doctors typically prescribe antibiotics to treat any underlying infections. They may also need to perform surgical revascularization to address restricted blood flow to the area. Your doctor may also remove any calluses and dead or infected tissue. In extreme cases, removal of bone or amputation of the foot may be necessary.

Venous ulcers

Venous ulcers are open sores that occur on the legs. They are the most common chronic leg ulcers, affecting 1–3% of people in the United States.

Causes

Two conditions that affect your veins typically cause venous ulcers are;

- Chronic venous insufficiency: This means that your leg veins are not returning blood to the heart effectively.

- Venous hypertension: This means that there is increased pressure in your veins.

These conditions cause excess blood to build up in your leg veins, increasing the pressure and causing an ulcer to form.

Symptoms

Venous ulcers are typically irregular, shallow open wounds on the legs. They often form over bones, such as the lower leg bone or the ankle. The ulcers can have a brownish color, and they may have discharge.

Other symptoms of venous ulcers include a rash, pain, itchy skin, varicose veins, or veins that are twisted and enlarged, spider veins, which are twisted veins that are smaller than varicose veins, atrophie blanche, or a scar with a distinctive pattern or inflammation

Diagnosis

To diagnose venous ulcers, your doctor will examine the wound and the skin around it. They will assess the location of the wound and determine if there are signs of venous insufficiency. Like with arterial ulcers, a doctor may perform an ABPI test to check your blood pressure. They may also perform a color-flow duplex ultrasound, which will help them analyze your vein structure and blood flow.

Treatment

Treatment for venous ulcers typically falls into two categories.

- Compression therapy: This involves using hosiery or bandages to apply gentle pressure to the leg, which will promote better blood flow.

- Wound care: Keeping the wound clean and avoiding infection is essential to promote healing.

In some cases, skin grafting may be necessary. Doctors may also need to perform endovenous ablation, which is a procedure that closes off varicose veins.

Genital ulcers

Genital ulcers are sores that appear on the genitals. Common locations include the penis, scrotum, anus, and vulva.

Causes

The main causes of genital ulcers are sexually transmitted infections (STIs). These include herpes simplex virus, syphilis, chlamydia or chancroid, which is a rare STI. Another cause of genital ulcers is Behçet's syndrome, which is a rare inflammatory condition. Genital ulcers caused by Behçet's syndrome typically occur on the penis, scrotum, or vulva.

Symptoms

The symptoms of genital ulcers will vary depending on which STI caused them. For example, the ulcer may appear as a single lesion, or there may be a cluster. Ulcers may or may not hurt or itch. It is also possible for you to develop a fever or feel generally unwell.

Diagnosis

To diagnose genital ulcers, doctors usually test for STIs. The results will help them determine the best treatment for you.

Treatment

Treatment for genital ulcers varies depending on the cause. Doctors may prescribe antiviral medications, antibiotics, or pain relievers.

Mouth ulcers

Mouth ulcers, or canker sores, occur inside your mouth. They can appear on your tongue or the inside of your cheeks or lips.

Causes

The causes of mouth ulcers include:

- trauma to the mouth, such as biting your cheek or having ill-fitting dentures or braces

- cuts or burns from eating or drinking

- a food allergy or intolerance

- hormonal changes

- an iron or vitamin B12 deficiency

- a weakened immune system

- certain conditions, such as Crohn's disease or celiac disease

- oral cancer

Symptoms

The symptoms of mouth ulcers usually include one or more sores inside your mouth that may change in size.

The sores may be painful, and the skin around them may look swollen.

Diagnosis

Doctors typically diagnose mouth ulcers by swabbing the ulcers to check for bacterial or viral infections. If you are feeling unwell, they may also perform blood tests. If your doctor suspects that cancer might be causing the ulcers, they may biopsy them. This procedure involves removing a piece of an ulcer for analysis in a laboratory.

Treatment

Treatment for mouth ulcers can include:

- applying topical corticosteroids or taking anti-inflammatory medications

- using antibiotic mouthwash

- avoiding foods that may worsen the ulcer

CHAPTER TWO

DIETING FOR ULCER

Your doctor may recommend making some dietary shifts to alleviate symptoms of stomach ulcers and to support healing. But what exactly should be on the menu depends on what triggers symptoms for you individually. With that ambiguity in mind, a generally healthy diet is considered best in supporting those with stomach ulcers. However, there are some food items that you might try eliminating or prioritizing to see what makes you feel better.

Certain foods and drinks can upset your stomach or increase stomach acid production, though there's not much evidence they can cause or worsen ulcers specifically. Still, because some food and beverage items can irritate your stomach, pay attention to how your body reacts.

Take spicy food, for instance. Everybody jumps right to spicy food (to eliminate). But what's interesting about that is that's not always the case. You have to see how it affects you; if spicy food bothers your stomach, avoid that particular food. But it's not necessarily completely off the menu, so to speak, for folks if they have a history of ulcers.

If you experience symptoms like burning pain in the middle or upper stomach, bloating after eating or increased heartburn after eating, that's a sign you should avoid a food.

You commonly avoided foods and beverages should include Alcohol, Acidic foods like pineapple, Citrus fruits, Spicy foods, Fatty or greasy foods, Pepper, including black pepper and other types of peppers, Caffeine, including caffeinated sodas, Tea, including black and green varieties that contain tannins, which can increase the production of stomach acid, Coffee, including decaf, Mint, including peppermint and spearmint, Spearmint, Chocolate, Carbonated beverages, Raw vegetables or salads and Tomatoes

One key element of your diet may be polyphenols, which are compounds found in fruits and vegetables that support digestion and brain health and provide other health benefits. Among the food items that could potentially prevent or even treat certain types of stomach ulcers, include Apples, Grapes, Pomegranates, Vegetables, Curcumin (a compound found in the bright orange spice turmeric), The leaves of the betel vine, which come from a family of plants indigenous to southern Asia that includes pepper and kava.

Similarly, eating plenty of fruits, vegetables and fiber because high consumption of produce, dietary fiber and vitamin A are associated with a reduced risk of ulcer disease.

Fiber, can also help ease constipation and decrease stomach acid. Sweet potatoes, for instance, may have some positive impact on stomach ulcers.

Alkaline foods can help provide relief from peptic ulcer symptoms as well. Alkaline and high-fiber foods include Watermelon, Bananas, Peaches, Apples, Pears, Broccoli, Avocado, Spinach, Kale, Potatoes, Soy,

Green beans, Lentils, Whole grains, Healthy fats, such as olive oil and avocado oil, Nuts, Fermented dairy products, such as yogurt, kefir and buttermilk, Fermented foods, such as sauerkraut, miso, kimchi and plant-based yogurts with active cultures.

And if you're having difficulty eating, opt for healthy foods that are high in calories to make sure you're meeting your energy needs. You may hurt when you eat, you may have cramps, you may have discomfort. But it's good to eat healthy, calorie-rich foods and small, frequent meals. Homemade shakes made with healthy ingredients, such as plant-based yogurt or ice cream, fruit, bananas, peanut butter and avocado, can help.

Foods with antibacterial or anti-inflammatory properties, such as honey and ginger, can also help support your body's ability to heal from an ulcer

Even thou there is no specific diet to follow to heal a peptic ulcer but have work my way around it and have come to a conclusion of some particular recipes you can diet with and you are good to go!

First, what you can do is find the foods that are right for you. As outlined earlier, avoid foods that exacerbate symptoms, such as those that boost stomach acid production. Second, prioritize fiber-, alkaline- and antioxidant-rich foods, which can lower acid production and help in the healing process. These two steps can help symptom management and support overall health.

Probiotics, the "good" bacteria that promotes the growth of protective gut microorganisms, can also play a key role in mitigating one of the causes of peptic ulcers: an H. pylori infection. A growing body of research, for instance, is showing that fermented foods, like those listed above, might inhibit the activity of H. pylori. While science still doesn't fully understand the connection between the gut microbiome and health, keep in mind that there's little evidence that probiotic supplements can help. That evidence is also limited to supplements' use when treating H. pylori bacterial infections. Certain strains of probiotics, however, may reduce diarrhea caused by the antibiotics used to treat H. pylori.

Also your lifestyle is important. Managing stress, getting proper rest and staying hydrated can aid in healing.

RECIPES FOR ULCER

Carrot and Kale Quinoa Patties
Total Time: 35 Mins

Ingredients

- olive oil

- 1½ cups cooked quinoa (equates to 1/2 cup uncooked quinoa)

- 2 tablespoons ground flaxseeds and 6 tablespoons of water, soaked for 10 minutes

- 1 cup kale, finely chopped (equates to approximately three leaves)

- 1/2 cup rolled oats, ground into flour (For a gluten-free patty, use gluten-free oats)

- 1/2 cup carrot, finely grated (equates to half of one large carrot)

- 1/4 cup pumpkin seeds

- 1/4 cup fresh basil, finely chopped

- 1/4 cup nutritional yeast

- 1/4 cup onion, finely diced

- equates to half a small onion

- 1 clove of garlic, minced

- 1 tablespoon tahini

- salt and pepper

Directions

- Preheat the oven to 400°F.

- Line a baking tray with baking paper.

- Heat the oil in a frying pan over a medium heat and cook the onions for five minutes or until soft. Add the garlic and cook for a further two minutes.

- Combine all ingredients, including the cooked onion and garlic, together in a large bowl. Stir well until the mixture comes together.

- With wet hands, shape mixture into 1/4 cup patties. Pack tightly so they will hold together better. Place onto lined baking tray.

- Bake for 15 minutes then turn and bake for a further 10 minutes or until golden.

- Allow to cool for 5 minutes then enjoy. Leftovers can be stored in the fridge to up to 5 days. Enjoy cold or to reheat, preheat a frying pan, and cook patties for about 3 minutes on each side in a little bit of oil.

Total Time: 56 Mins

Ingredients

- 1 tablespoon extra-virgin olive oil

- 1/2 medium yellow onion, chopped

- 1/2 teaspoon sea salt

- 3 garlic cloves, smashed

- 1 pound carrots, roughly chopped

- 1 teaspoon grated fresh ginger

- 1 tablespoon apple cider vinegar

- 3 cups vegetable broth

- freshly ground black pepper

- 1 teaspoon maple syrup, optional

- coconut milk for garnish, optional

Directions

- Heat the oil in a large pot over medium heat. Add the onions, salt and pepper and cook until softened, stirring occasionally, about 8 minutes. Add the smashed garlic cloves (they'll get blended later) and carrots to the pot and cook 8 minutes more, stirring occasionally.

- Stir in the ginger, apple cider vinegar, and broth. Bring to a boil, then reduce the heat and simmer for 30 minutes.

- Let cool slightly and transfer to a blender. Blend until smooth. If your soup is too thick, add a little water. If you would like your soup a little sweeter, add the maple syrup.

- Serve with a drizzle of coconut milk, if desired.

Total Time: 40 Mins

Ingredients

- 1 cup uncooked quinoa, rinsed in a fine-mesh colander

- 2 cups water

- 1 can (15 ounces) chickpeas, rinsed and drained, or 1 ½ cups cooked chickpeas

- 1 medium cucumber, seeded and chopped

- 1 medium red bell pepper, chopped

- ¾ cup chopped red onion (from 1 small red onion)

- 1 cup finely chopped flat-leaf parsley (from 1 large bunch)

- ¼ cup olive oil

- ¼ cup lemon juice (from 2 to 3 lemons)

- 1 tablespoon red wine vinegar

- 2 cloves garlic, pressed or minced

- ½ teaspoon fine sea salt

- Freshly ground black pepper, to taste

Directions

- Combine the rinsed quinoa and the water in a medium saucepan. Bring the mixture to a boil over medium-high heat, then decrease the heat to maintain a gentle simmer. Cook, uncovered, until the quinoa has absorbed all of the water, about 15 minutes, reducing heat as time goes on to maintain a gentle simmer. Remove from heat, cover, and let the quinoa rest for 5 minutes, to give it time to fluff up.

- In a large serving bowl, combine the chickpeas, cucumber, bell pepper, onion and parsley. Set aside.

- In a small bowl, combine the olive oil, lemon juice, vinegar, garlic and salt. Whisk until blended, then set aside.

- Once the quinoa is mostly cool, add it to the serving bowl, and drizzle the dressing on top. Toss until the mixture is thoroughly combined. Season with black pepper, to taste, and add an extra pinch of salt if necessary. For best flavor, let the salad rest for 5 to 10 minutes before serving.

Fresh Cranberry Scones

Total Time: 40 Mins

Ingredients

- 1 package fresh cranberries, minimum 6 ounces, maximum 12 ounces

- 1/3 cup brown sugar, not packed

- 2 1/4 cups AP flour

- 3 teaspoons baking powder

- 1/2 teaspoon salt

- zest of 2 organic oranges

- 1/4 chopped candied ginger

- 10 tablespoons chilled coconut oil, cut into small pieces

- 1/3 soy/almond milk

Directions

- Preheat oven 350ºF and line baking sheet with parchment paper.

- In food processor, pulse the cranberries with the brown sugar and orange zest. go for chunky. put in large mixing bowl, set aside.

- In food processor, pulse the AP flower, baking powder and salt. add in the coconut oil and pulse until pea-sized crumbles appear.

- Mix the flour mixture with the cranberries in the mixing bowl. add the milk and stir until it just comes together.

- Dust counter with a bit of flour, dump dough onto it. form a disk/thick circle. cut into quarters, and within those quarters cut 3 wedges.

- Carefully transfer wedges on prepared baking sheet and bake for 40-45 minutes, rotating the baking sheet half way through.

- The edges and bottom will darken a little, but the interior will be tender and crumbly.

- Serve warm, as is, or drizzled with icing (you can make a quick icing slurry of 2 teaspoons the milk used plus enough powdered sugar to get a thickened but drizzly consistency, anywhere from 10-15 tablespoons).

Blueberry Pancakes with Blueberry-Maple Syrup

Total Time: 25 Mins

Ingredients

- 1½ cups all purpose flour, spooned into measuring cup and leveled off

- 2 tablespoons sugar

- 2½ teaspoons baking powder

- ½ teaspoon salt

- 1 small, over-ripe banana, peeled (the browner, the better)

- 2 large eggs

- 1 cup plus 2 tablespoons low fat milk

- ½ teaspoon vanilla extract

- 3 tablespoons unsalted butter, melted

- 1 - 2 tablespoons vegetable oil

- 1 tablespoon unsalted butter

Directions

- In a medium bowl, whisk together the flour, sugar, baking powder and salt.

- In a small bowl, mash the banana with a fork until almost smooth. Whisk in the eggs, then add the milk and vanilla and whisk until well blended. Pour the banana mixture and the melted butter into the flour mixture. Fold the batter gently with a rubber spatula until just blended; do not over-mix. The batter will be thick and lumpy.

- Set a griddle or non-stick pan over medium heat until hot. Put a pad of butter and one tablespoon vegetable oil onto the griddle, and swirl it around. Drop the batter by ¼-cupfuls onto the griddle, spacing the pancakes about 2 inches apart. Cook until a few holes form on top of each pancake and the underside is golden brown, about 2 minutes. Flip the pancakes and cook until the bottom is golden brown and the top is puffed, 1 to 2 minutes more. Using the spatula, transfer the pancakes to a serving plate.

- Wipe the griddle clean with paper towels, add more butter and oil, and repeat with the remaining batter. Serve the pancakes while still hot with maple syrup, sliced bananas and confectioners' sugar if desired.

- The pancakes can be frozen for up to 3 months. After they are completely cooled, place a sheet of parchment or wax paper between each pancake and stack together. Wrap the stack of pancakes tightly in aluminum foil or place inside a heavy-duty freezer bag. To reheat, place them in a single layer on a baking sheet and cover with foil. Bake in a 375°F oven for about 8 to 10 minutes, or until hot.

Quinoa Berry Breakfast Bowl

Total Time: 15 Mins

Ingredients

- 1 cup cooked quinoa

- ½ cup strawberries, hulled and sliced

- ½ cup raspberries, rinsed

- ½ cup blueberries, rinsed

- ½ cup blackberries, rinsed

- ¼ cup sliced almonds

- 1 tablespoon hemp or flax seeds

- 1 teaspoon maple syrup

- ¼ cup of light coconut milk, shaken

Directions

- Cook quinoa and allow to cool. Prepare mixed berries.

- Pour all the ingredients into a medium-sized bowl, ending with the coconut milk. Stir gently. Serve in cereal bowls.

Spinach & Mushroom Egg Muffins
Total Time: 30 Mins

Ingredients

- Olive oil spray, 1 x two-second spray(s)

- Extra virgin olive oil, 1 tsp(s)

- Mushrooms, 1½ cup(s), slices

- Red onion, chopped, ¼ cup(s)

- Baby spinach, 2 cup(s), roughly chopped

- Eggs, 5 large

- 1% milk, 3 tbsp(s)

- Black pepper, 3 dash(es)

- Cheddar cheese, reduced-fat, shredded, 4 tbsp(s)

Directions

- Preheat the oven to 350°F. Spray 8 holes of a 12-cup muffin pan with oil or use muffin tin liners.

- Heat the oil in a non-stick skillet over medium-low heat. Add the mushrooms and onion and cook while stirring, until soft, about 5 to 10 minutes. Add the spinach and cook until wilted. Remove from heat.

- Divide mushroom mixture evenly between the 8 muffin cups.

- In a medium bowl, whisk the eggs, milk and black pepper. Pour in the egg mixture to evenly cover the vegetables and top with the cheese. Bake for 18 to 20 minutes.

Total Time: 30 Mins

Ingredients

- ¼ cup olive oil

- ¼ cup lemon juice

- zest of 1 lemon

- 2-3 garlic clove crushed

- 2 tsp fresh thyme

- 2 tsp rosemary

- 1 tsp dried oregano

- 1 tsp salt

- 1 tsp pepper

- For the skewers

- 4 large chicken breasts skinless, boneless

- wooden skewers soaked in boiling water for 30 minutes

Directions

- Combine all the ingredients for the marinade.

- Slice the chicken into bite-sized chunks and place in a bowl. Pour over the marinade, cover and allow to marinade for at least 30 minutes but up to 24 hours, covered in the fridge.

- Thread the marinated chicken onto soaked wooden skewers or metal skewers.

- Heat an outdoor grill or stovetop grill pan then cook the skewers, turning every 3-5 minutes, until the chicken is cooked through and golden brown on all sides.

- Remove from the heat and allow to rest for 5 minutes before serving.

Total Time: 25 Mins

Ingredients

- ¼ cup olive oil

- ¼ cup lemon juice

- zest of 1 lemon

- 2-3 garlic clove crushed

- 2 tsp fresh thyme

- 2 tsp rosemary

- 1 tsp dried oregano

- 1 tsp salt

- 1 tsp pepper

- 4 large chicken breasts skinless, boneless

- wooden skewers soaked in boiling water for 30 minutes

Directions

- Combine all the ingredients for the marinade.

- Slice the chicken into bite-sized chunks and place in a bowl. Pour over the marinade, cover and allow to marinade for at least 30 minutes but up to 24 hours, covered in the fridge.

- Thread the marinated chicken onto soaked wooden skewers or metal skewers.

- Heat an outdoor grill or stovetop grill pan then cook the skewers, turning every 3-5 minutes, until the chicken is cooked through and golden brown on all sides.

- Remove from the heat and allow to rest for 5 minutes before serving.

Cheese and vegetable omelette

Total Time: 25 Mins

Ingredients

- 1 scallion, diced

- 1/2 medium red pepper, deseeded and diced

- 3 button mushrooms, sliced

- 2 medium eggs

- 20g / 1oz. of low-fat cheese, grated

- 1 serving of spinach (90g / 3oz.), roughly chopped

- ½ tomato, sliced

- Black pepper, to taste

- 1 slice of wholemeal bread, toasted

- 1 teaspoon of low-fat spread

- Spray a small non-stick pan with cooking spray and heat over a medium heat

Directions

- Add the scallion, pepper and mushrooms and cook for 5 minutes until the vegetables begin to soften.

- Crack the eggs in a bowl and combine with the grated cheese, spinach, tomato and a little black pepper to taste.

- When the vegetables in the pan are ready, add to the egg mixture, mix well and return to the pan.

- Cook the omelette for 2-3 minutes, until the edges cook and come away from the edge of the pan, the mixture should be firm. If you do not want to flip the omelette, preheat your grill.

- To finish your omelette, either finish under the grill for another minute, or flip in the pan and leave to cook for the same amount of time.

- Optional: As you finish cooking your omelette, toast the bread to have ready to enjoy together

Garlic Sautéed Spinach

Total Time: 10 Mins

Ingredients

- 1 pound baby spinach

- 2 tablespoons olive oil

- 3 garlic cloves, minced

- salt and pepper, to taste

Directions

- Heat the olive oil in a large skillet over medium-high heat. Add the minced garlic and saute for 30 seconds. You don't want the garlic browning too much.

- Heating garlic and oil in a pan for garlic sauteed spinach.

- Add the baby spinach to the pan. It will be a big mound, and you can use your hands to pack it in. Use tongs or a spatula to carefully flip the spinach over, so that all of the pieces get covered in oil and garlic.

- Cover the pan for a minute to let it steam, then stir again. Repeat this process until the spinach is wilted down, about 5 minutes later.

- Covering a pan of garlic sauteed spinach for steaming.

- Season with salt and pepper, then serve.

Healthy Ground Turkey Stir Fry
Total Time: 30 Mins

Ingredients

- 3 tablespoons olive oil, plus more if necessary

- 1 to 2 tablespoons sesame oil, or as desired

- 1 large sweet Vidalia onion, diced small

- 1 pound ground turkey (ground chicken, ground pork sausage, or ground beef may be substituted)

- 1 orange bell pepper, seeded and diced small

- 1 yellow bell pepper, seeded and diced small

- 1 1/2 cups baby carrots, halved

- 1/3 cup reduced-sodium soy sauce, or as desired

- 1 to 2 tablespoons chili garlic sauce, or as desired (start with 1 teaspoon if you're sensitive to heat and work up from there)

- 1 large zucchini, diced into bite-sized piece

- 1 broccoli crown, diced into bite-sized florets

- kosher salt and freshly ground black pepper, to taste

Directions

- To a large and high-sided skillet, add the oils, onion, and saute over medium-high heat for about 4 minutes, or until onion is beginning to soften; stir frequently.

- Add the turkey, peppers, carrots, and cook over medium-high heat for about 7 minutes, or until turkey is cooked through and vegetables are crisp-tender. Crumble and stir the turkey as it cooks to ensure even cooking.

- Add the soy sauce, chili garlic sauce, and stir to incorporate evenly.

- Add the zucchini, broccoli, stir to combine, and cover the skillet with a lid to encourage the broccoli to steam. Cook for about 3 minutes, or until broccoli is as tender as desired.

- Season with salt and pepper to taste and serve immediately.

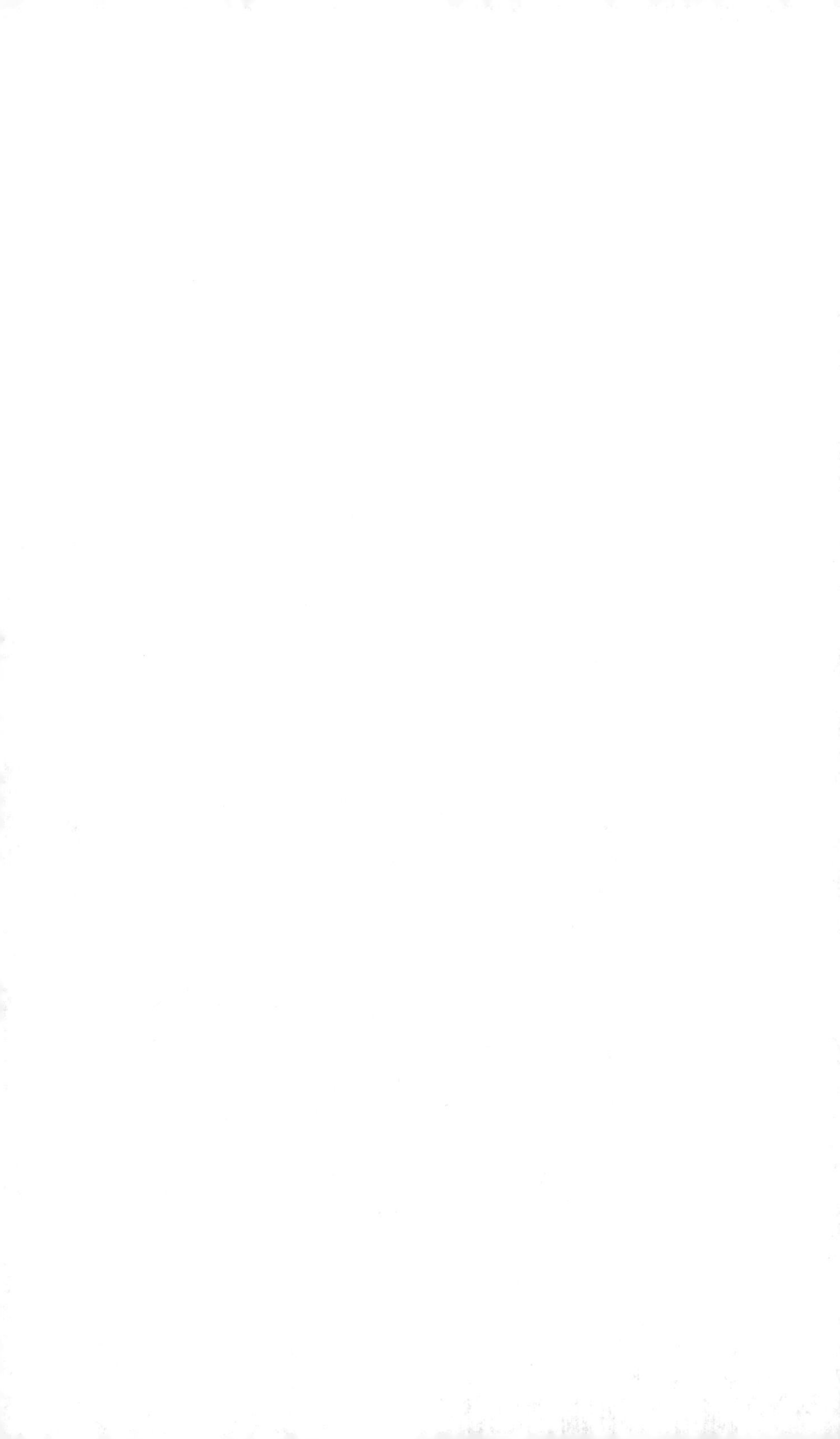